AGELESS AT 50:

A Guide to Achieving Optimal Health and Vitality

THIS
BOOK
BELONG
TO

____

____

Table of Contents

INTRODUCTION OF THE IMPORTANCE OF LOOKING AND FEELING HEALTHY AT 50.

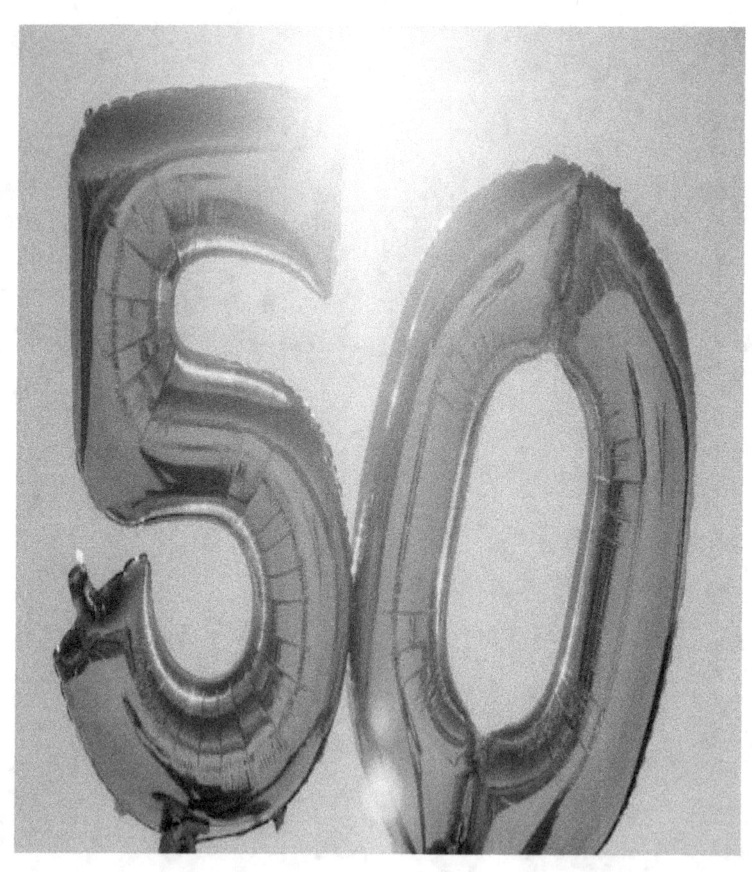

When people cross the 50-year-old mark, maintaining good looks and physical health becomes quite important. During this phase of life, which is frequently characterized by change, a person's physical and mental health have a big influence on their lifespan, general quality of life, and capacity to enjoy the rewards of their hard work. We will examine the strong arguments for why it is crucial to look and feel good at 50 in this introduction.

1. Improved Quality of Life: Living a more contented and pleasurable life at 50 can be facilitated by maintaining good health. It permits people to keep a high degree of freedom, pursue their interests, and be active. A healthy lifestyle is the cornerstone of an enriched existence, whether it involves travel, socializing with loved ones, or engaging in hobbies.

2. Longevity: Longevity and health are closely

related. People can raise their odds of living longer and more vibrant lives by adopting a healthy lifestyle and making wise decisions. Because it gives them more time to spend with their loved ones, this helps not just the individual but also them.

3. Physical Fitness: Preventing age-related health problems requires maintaining physical fitness at 50. Frequent exercise maintains bone density, joint flexibility, and muscular mass. It is also essential in lowering the chance of developing long-term illnesses like diabetes, hypertension, and heart disease.

4. Mental Well-Being: Physical and mental well-being are interdependent. At fifty, feeling well can help with improved mental clarity, emotional balance, and a lower chance of developing mental health issues like anxiety and depression. A fulfilling existence in older years requires both emotional fortitude and mental acuity.

5. Social and Emotional Relationships: One's confidence and sense of self-worth can be greatly impacted by their physical health and looks. At fifty, having good health can increase self-confidence and facilitate the establishment and upkeep of social and emotional connections. Longevity and happiness are correlated with strong social ties.

6. Financial Considerations: Illness might result in a loss of income and substantial healthcare bills. People who prioritize their health at 50 may be able to save money on medical costs and carry on with their jobs or favorite hobbies.

7. Providing a Good Example: Maintaining good health at 50 leaves a lasting impression on future generations. It promotes a healthier society by highlighting the value of leading a healthy lifestyle and inspiring kids and grandkids to follow suit. In conclusion, it is critical to maintain a good appearance and sense of well-being beyond 50. It improves the person's quality of life and has a positive knock-on effect on their loved ones and the community as a whole. People can welcome this milestone with energy and grace and take advantage of all the benefits that come with aging well if they have the correct attitude, lifestyle choices, and access to healthcare services.

1. CHAPTER

EMBRACING THE AGE OF 50

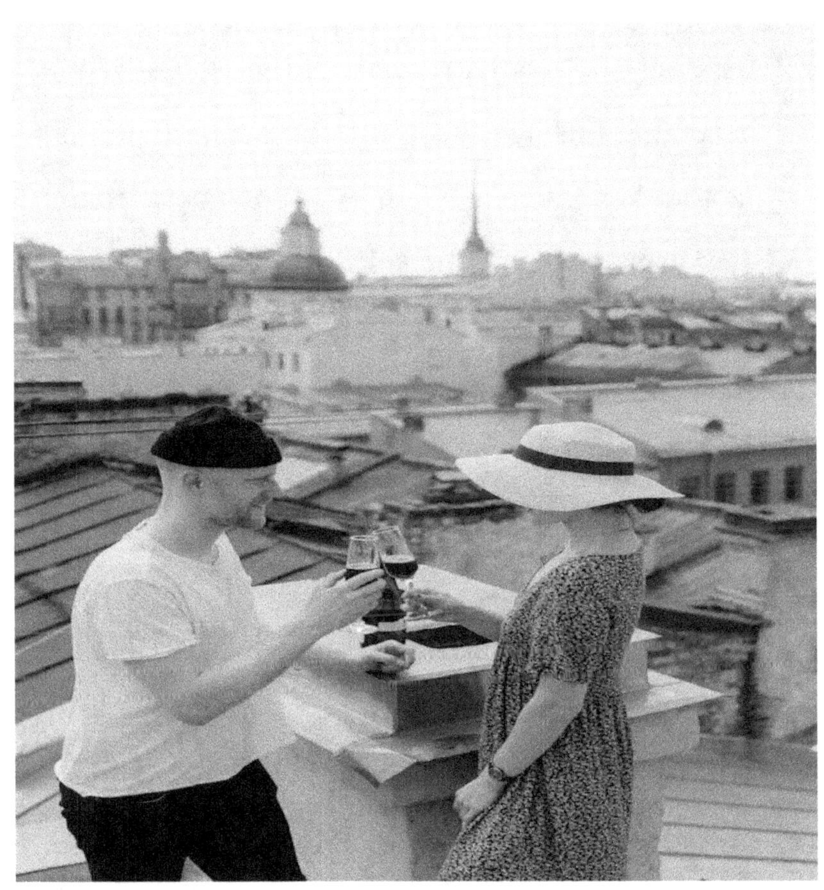

Reaching fifty is a powerful and life-changing turning point in one's path. At this point in time, people are standing at the nexus of history and the future, having amassed a multitude of experiences, insights, and life lessons. While accepting this age, keep the following important factors in mind:

1. Acceptance of Oneself: Reaching fifty is a chance to accept and truly embrace oneself, flaws and all. Now is the perfect moment to let go of illusory expectations and appreciate the beauty of being who you are.

2. Reflection: Give yourself some time to consider the path that has led you here. Honor your successes and draw lessons from your setbacks. Thinking back on the past might provide you important insights for the future.

3. Creating New Objectives: While acknowledging previous successes, it's critical to create new objectives and aspirations for the future. Setting objectives can provide life direction and excitement, whether they are related to professional aspirations, personal development, or vacation experiences.

4. Wellness and Health: Give your mental and physical well-being first priority. At this age, preventative healthcare measures, a balanced diet, and regular exercise become more crucial. Seeking medical guidance and testing to make sure you're on the proper road shouldn't be discouraged.

5. Lifelong Learning: Accept that there is always more to learn. Keep learning new things, taking up new interests, and broadening your horizons. This gives your life more depth and keeps your mind active.

6. Financial Planning: Review your retirement and financial objectives. To make sure you're on a safe financial route for the future, get financial advice if needed.

7. Relationships: Take care of and treasure your bonds with loved ones and friends. Keeping meaningful relationships becomes even more crucial for mental health when life gets busier.

8. Travel and Adventure: Take into account seeing and doing new things. Traveling opens your mind, makes memories that last a lifetime, and gives you a sense of adventure that keeps life interesting.

9. Giving Back: Giving back to the communities or causes they are passionate about brings fulfillment to many people. Giving back to the community and volunteering can give one a sense of fulfillment and purpose.

10. Mindfulness and Gratitude: Consistently cultivate gratitude and mindfulness. Spend some time appreciating the here and now and expressing your thanks for the people and things in your life that have made it better.

11. Adaptability: Be open to change and be flexible. At fifty, life may take you in unexpected directions, but you may grow and become resilient by being open to new opportunities.

12. Self-Care: Make self-care a priority. This includes finding peaceful and joyful activities as well as ways to decompress and handle stress. Essentially, accepting oneself at the age of fifty means appreciating the depth of one's life's experience, past and present. This is the time to live intentionally, make decisions that reflect your goals and ideals, and cherish the important moments in life. You can enter the next stage of your life with grace and passion if you approach this age with a good outlook and a dedication to your health.

2. CHAPTER

Understanding the Aging Process

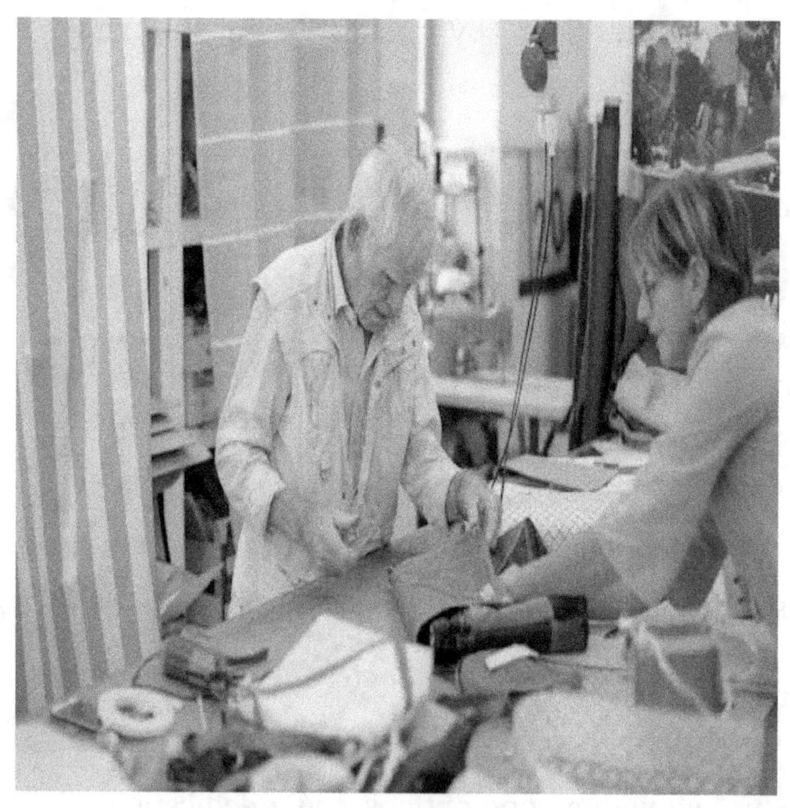

For both people and society at large, understanding the aging process is crucial. Aging is a biological phenomenon that is complex, natural, and unavoidable that impacts all living things, including humans. Numerous alterations in the physical, psychological, and social domains are involved. This is a thorough rundown of the main elements of the aging process:

1. Biological Aging:

- **Cellular Senescence**: The body's cells change with time, affecting how they operate. This includes a reduction in their capacity for self-healing and an increase in the synthesis of toxic compounds.

The protective caps on the ends of chromosomes called telomeres shorten with every cell division. Aging results from cells that are unable to divide when they get too short.

- **Hormonal Changes:** As people age, their bodies produce less growth hormone and sex hormones, which can cause a variety of physiological and physical changes.

- **Strength and Muscle Mass:** As muscle mass tends to decline, so does physical endurance and strength.

2. Physical Changes:

- **Bone density:** As bone density declines, people become more prone to osteoporosis and fractures.

- **Skin Changes:** Skin becomes more prone to wrinkles and age spots, grows thinner, and loses its elastic properties.

- Age-related changes in vision, hearing, taste, and smell are examples of sensory changes.

3. Cognitive Changes:

- **Memory:** It's common to experience some age-related memory loss, especially when it comes to recalling specific facts. On the other hand, severe memory loss may indicate cognitive diseases such as dementia.

- **Processing Speed:** As one ages, their ability to process information may diminish.

- **Wisdom and Expertise:** Senior citizens frequently have a plethora of knowledge and experience, which improves their capacity for problem-solving and making decisions.

4. Psychological Changes: Emotional Regulation: As people age, their capacity to regulate their emotions may improve, resulting in increased emotional stability and resilience.

- **Psychological Well-Being:** Senior citizens may express greater levels of contentment and life satisfaction.

- **Social Networks:** People's social circles can alter due to retirement, moving, or losing loved ones. Sustaining social relationships becomes more crucial for mental and emotional health.

5. Social Shifts:

Retirement may present chances for relaxation and exploring individual passions, but it might also necessitate monetary modifications and a change in daily schedules.

Chronic Conditions: As one ages, there is an increased chance of developing chronic illnesses like cancer, diabetes, and heart disease.

6. Health Challenges:

Medication: In order to treat these illnesses, older persons may need to take several medications, which might result in polypharmacy and possible adverse effects.ϖ

7. Lifestyle Factors:

Diet and Exercise: Eating a well-balanced diet and getting regular exercise helps lessen the negative effects of aging on the body and mind.

Mental Stimulation: Solving puzzles, reading, or picking up new skills are examples of cognitively demanding activities that might improve cognitive health.

- **Positive Attitude:** Having a positive view on aging can help improve both mental and physical health.v

8. Attitude and Adaptability:

- **Adaptability:** Aging gracefully requires the capacity to accept new experiences and adjust to changing circumstances. People who are aware of the aging process are more equipped to make decisions as they age regarding their lifestyle, health, and general well-being. It also helps researchers, politicians, and healthcare professionals create plans to support healthy aging and deal with the problems brought on by an aging population.

3. CHAPTER

THE ROLE OF NUTRITION

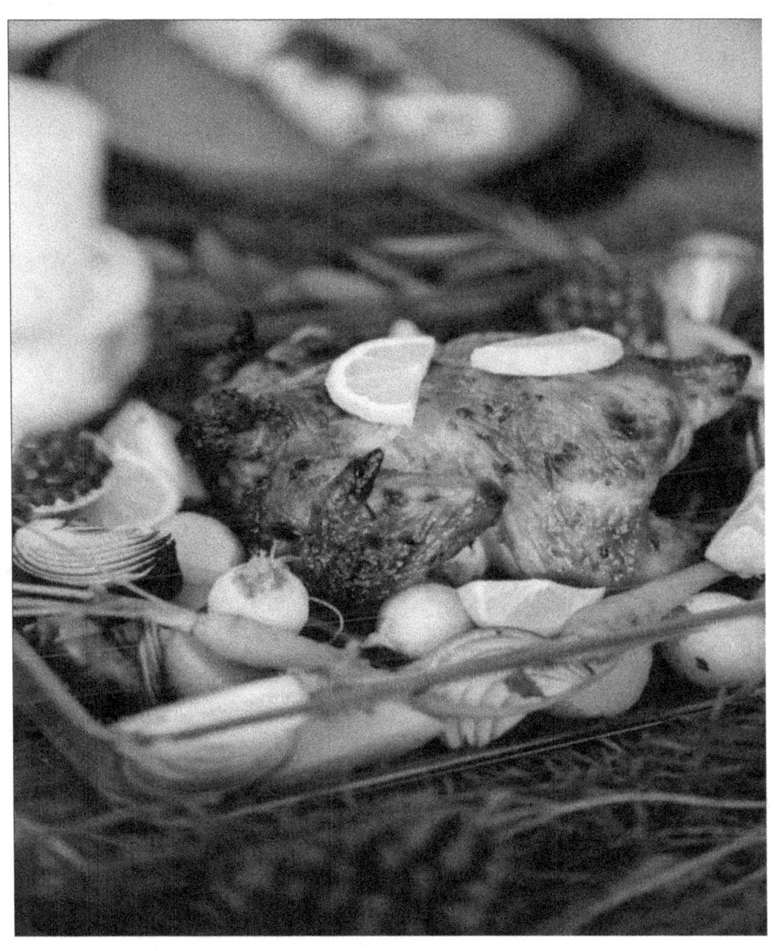

As people age, diet plays a more and more important role, especially for those over the age of 50. Maintaining excellent health, preventing chronic diseases, fostering physical and emotional well-being, and extending life expectancy are all greatly influenced by proper nutrition. The following are important facets of how diet affects aging:

1. **Physical Health:**

- **Bone and muscular Health:** Sustaining muscular mass and strength requires consuming enough protein. Osteoporosis, which becomes problematic as people age, can be avoided by maintaining bone density and taking vitamin D and calcium supplements.ϖ1. Physical Health: Heart Health: Eating a diet reduced in sodium, trans fats, and saturated fats will help lower the risk of hypertension and heart disease. Foods high in fiber can also help control cholesterol levels.

Digestive Health: Fiber from whole grains, fruits, and vegetables helps encourage regular bowel movements and stave off constipation, which is a major problem among older persons.

2. Chronic Disease Prevention: Diabetes Management: Blood sugar levels can be controlled, particularly for people who have diabetes or are at risk, by keeping an eye on carbohydrate intake and selecting complex carbs.

- **Cancer Prevention:** Consuming a diet high in antioxidant-rich fruits and vegetables helps lower the chance of developing some cancers.

- **Managing Weight:** Eating a balanced diet that keeps you at a healthy weight helps avoid or control obesity, which is connected to a number of chronic conditions.

3. Cognitive Health

Brain Health: Certain vitamins and minerals (e.g., vitamin E, omega-3 fatty acids) and antioxidants are linked to cognitive health and may help lower the risk of neurodegenerative illnesses like Alzheimer's and cognitive decline.

Hydration: Maintaining proper hydration is crucial for cognitive performance, since dehydration can cause disorientation and decreased focus.

4. Mental Health:

Omega-3 Fatty Acids: These fats, which can be found in walnuts, flaxseeds, and fatty fish, may improve mood and lower the chance of developing depression.

- **B vitamins:** Sufficient consumption of B vitamins, specifically B6, B9 (folate), and B12, is critical for cognitive and mental well-being.

5. Immune Function:

- **Micronutrients:** Minerals and vitamins that strengthen the immune system, including zinc, selenium, vitamin C, and vitamin D, can help older persons maintain their health.

6. Gut Health:

- **Probiotics and Prebiotics:** Eating foods high in probiotics (yogurt, for example) and prebiotics (garlic, onions) might support a favorable gut microbiome, which is related to immunological and general health

7. Hydration:

Water Intake: Maintaining adequate hydration is essential for good health since dehydration can aggravate a number of conditions, such as urinary tract infections.

8. Medication Management: Certain drugs may have an impact on metabolism or nutrient absorption. It's crucial that senior citizens and their healthcare professionals talk about any possible nutritional interactions.

9. Social and Emotional Well-Being:

 Social Eating: Eating meals with loved ones can foster emotional support and social connection, which improves general wellbeing.

10. Individualized Nutrition Plans: Depending on variables including gender, degree of exercise, and underlying medical issues, older persons' nutritional needs might differ significantly. Consulting

4. CHAPTER

EXERCISE AND FITNESS

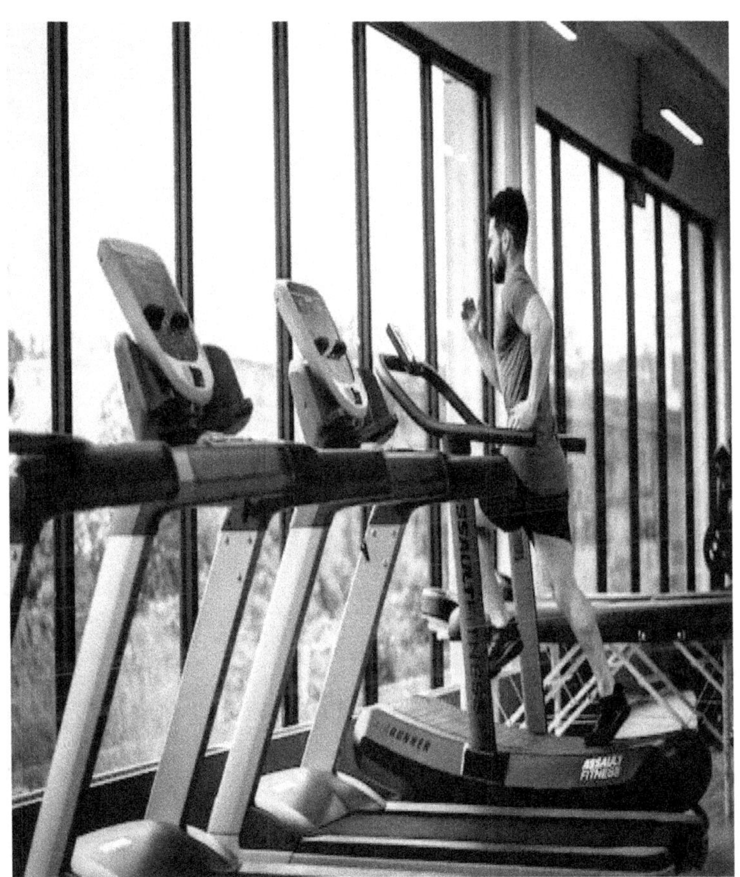

A healthy lifestyle is essentially centered around exercise and fitness, which become increasingly important as people age. This is particularly valid for people over 50. Numerous physical, mental, and emotional advantages of regular exercise improve one's general health and quality of life. This is an examination of how fitness and exercise affect aging:

1. Physical Health:

- **Muscle and Bone Health:** Exercise, especially weight-bearing exercises and resistance training, helps preserve bone density and muscle mass, which lowers the risk of osteoporosis and age-related muscle loss (sarcopenia).

- **Cardiovascular Health:** By enhancing cardiovascular fitness, lowering blood pressure, and lowering the risk of heart disease, aerobic exercise—such as brisk walking, jogging, or cycling—supports heart health.

- **Joint Mobility and Flexibility:** Frequent flexibility and stretching exercises can improve joint mobility and lower the chance of age-related stiffness and injury.

2. Weight Management: By burning calories and increasing lean muscle mass, exercise can help control body weight when combined with a healthy diet. Preventing obesity and its associated health problems is crucial.

3. Prevention and Management of Chronic Diseases: Exercise lowers the chance of developing long-term illnesses such as type 2 diabetes, hypertension, and several types of cancer. Exercise can assist people with chronic diseases manage their symptoms and enhance their general health.

4. Cognitive Health: Exercise encourages the release of neurotransmitters and growth factors that support brain health. Regular exercise has been related to cognitive advantages, including increased memory, enhanced cognitive function, and a decreased risk of cognitive decline and dementia.

5. Mental and Emotional Well-Being: Physical activity can increase self-esteem and confidence, which can result in a more optimistic attitude on life. Exercise also has a dramatic effect on mental health because it triggers the production of endorphins, which can reduce stress, anxiety, and depression.

6. Sleep Quality: Frequent physical activity can enhance sleep patterns and quality, which is crucial for general health and cognitive performance.

7. Energy and Vitality: Engaging in regular exercise improves stamina, boosts energy levels, and supports people in leading active, satisfying lives.

8. Social connection: Team sports and group

exercise programs offer chances for social connection and a sense of community, which can help fight feelings of loneliness and isolation, particularly in older persons.

9. Balance and Fall Prevention: Balance-focused exercises, including tai chi and yoga, can lower the risk of falls and increase general stability, which is crucial for older persons.

10. Longevity: Exercising regularly has been linked to a longer life expectancy, which enables people to live longer, more active, and meaningful lives.

11. Adaptability and Variety: People's fitness requirements and capacities may vary as they get older. To keep things fresh, it's critical to modify workout regimens to account for these shifts and experiment with different types of physical activity.

12. Consulting Healthcare Professionals: To guarantee safety and appropriateness, it's imperative to speak with a healthcare provider or a competent fitness expert before starting any exercise program, especially for individuals with pre-existing health concerns.

To sum up, fitness and exercise are essential for good aging. Engaging in regular physical activity can improve mental and physical health, lower the risk of chronic illnesses, and help people live vibrant, meaningful lives well into the age of fifty. Including exercise in daily activities is a proactive step toward living a high-quality senior years.

Was this a better or worse response?

5. chapter

MANAGING STRESS AND MENTAL HEALTH

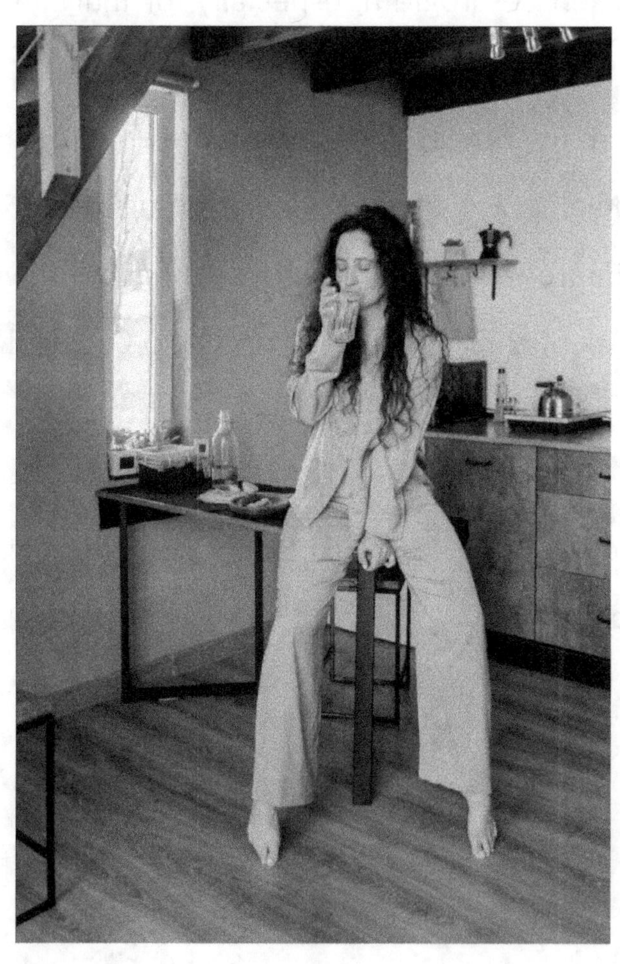

At every stage of life, stress management and mental health are critical, but as people age 50 and beyond, they become much more so. Particular difficulties may arise during this time, such as adjustments to one's lifestyle, health issues, and shifting circumstances. Here are some methods for handling stress and preserving mental well-being throughout this stage of life:

1. Remain Active: Engaging in regular physical activity promotes both mental and physical health. Exercise releases endorphins, which are naturally occurring mood boosters. Depending on one's fitness level and any physical restrictions, gentle yet effective activities like yoga, walking, or swimming can be chosen.

2. Mindfulness and Meditation: These two practices can lessen stress and enhance mental clarity. These methods encourage living in the now, which is particularly beneficial for controlling future-focused anxiety.

3. Social Connections: Keeping up and fostering social ties is essential to mental wellness. Participate in social events on a regular basis, maintain relationships with loved ones, and think about joining organizations or social groups based on your interests.

4. Seek Professional Assistance: Do not wait to get professional assistance if you are exhibiting signs of stress, anxiety, or depression. Mental health specialists, such therapists or counselors, can offer direction and assistance catered to your individual need.

5. Eating Well: A nutrient-dense, well-balanced diet has a good effect on mental and emotional well-being. Walnuts, flaxseeds, and seafood are good sources of omega-3 fatty acids, which have been related to better mental health. Stabilizing mood can also be achieved by consuming less sugar, caffeine, and processed foods.

6. Sufficient Sleep: Give proper sleep hygiene top priority. Make sure you obtain adequate restorative sleep every night because insufficient sleep can worsen stress and have a detrimental impact on mental health.

7. Time management: Plan out your everyday tasks and obligations to lessen the stress that comes with deadlines. Set reasonable goals and prioritize your tasks to prevent feeling overburdened.

8. Retirement Planning: If you are going to retire soon or have already done so, think about how you will organize your time and come to terms with this new stage of your life. Retirement might present a chance for pursuit of long-held hobbies and personal development.

9. Interests and Hobbies: Pursuing interests and hobbies that you are enthusiastic about might help you feel content and unwind. This can involve learning a new instrument, painting, or gardening, among other things.

10. Support Networks: Look for organizations that address your particular needs or interests or join support groups. Talking about difficulties and experiences with like-minded people can be quite helpful.

11. Minimize Stressors: Determine the causes of your stress and take action to lessen or get rid of them. This can entail making adjustments to your daily schedule, establishing limits, or asking for assistance when faced with daunting responsibilities.

12. Positive Thinking: Make an effort to think positively and to be kind to yourself. Refute negative thought patterns and concentrate on your accomplishments and strong points.

13. Expert Advice: To ensure you have a safe financial plan in place for the future and lessen financial stress, speak with retirement planners or financial consultants.

14. Remain Informed: Learn about the aging process and any potential medical issues. Anxiety over the unknown might be lessened by knowing what to expect.

15. provide Back and Volunteer: Volunteering or making charitable contributions can provide one a sense of fulfillment and purpose that can improve mental health. Recall that preserving mental health and controlling stress are continuous processes. Prioritizing self-care, getting help when you need it, and taking proactive measures to deal with stressors are crucial for leading a happy and psychologically sound life as you become older.

6. CHAPTER

SKINCARE AND GROOMING

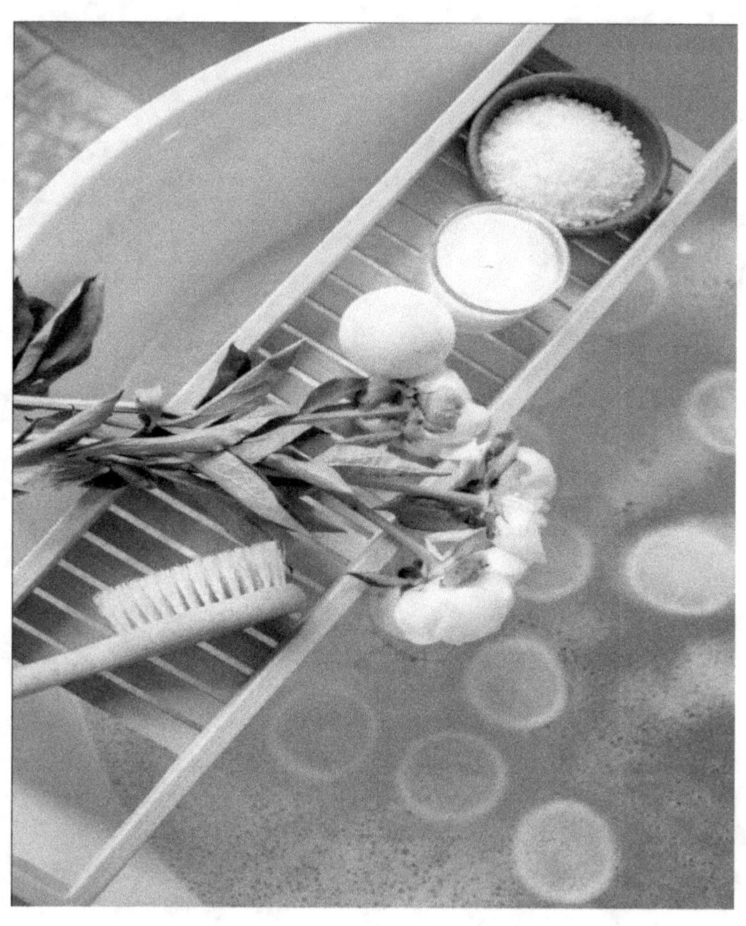

of self-care that grow more significant as people age 50 and beyond. Good grooming and skincare practices can support youthful appearance, good skin maintenance, and increased self-confidence. In your 50s and beyond, take into account the following advice and suggestions for skincare and grooming:

Skincare:

1. Daily Cleaning: Use a mild, moisturizing cleanser to wash your face twice a day in order to get rid of makeup, oil, and debris. Steer clear of strong or drying cleansers as they might remove natural oils from the skin.

2. Moisturize: To keep your skin supple and fight off dryness, which can become more common as you age, use a rich, moisturizing moisturizer. Keep an eye out for products that contain ceramides, glycerin, and hyaluronic acid.

3. Sun Protection: Even on overcast days, don't stop using sunscreen every day. In order to avoid age spots, wrinkles, and sun damage, use sunscreen. Pick a sunscreen that is broad-spectrum and has at least 30 SPF.

4. Exfoliation: To get rid of dead skin cells and encourage cell turnover, exfoliate your skin once or twice a week. For a mild exfoliation, think about utilizing chemical exfoliants like beta hydroxy acids (BHAs) or alpha hydroxy acids (AHAs).

5. Serums: Include anti-aging serums in your skincare regimen that contain retinol, vitamin C, and peptides. These may lessen the visibility of wrinkles and fine lines.

6. Eye Cream: To take care of the sensitive skin around the eyes, use a hydrating eye cream. For the treatment of aging symptoms like puffiness and dark circles, look for components like hyaluronic acid and peptides.

7. Night Cream: To heal and renew your skin while you sleep, use a nutritious night cream that contains components including antioxidants and hydrating agents.

8. Hydration: Drink lots of water to stay well-hydrated, as this can support both general health and skin hydration. Maintaining grooming

1. Haircare: To keep your hair clean and healthy, follow a regular haircare regimen that includes shampooing and conditioning. Think about getting a haircut that accentuates the features of your face and fits your lifestyle.

2. Hair Color: For the most natural-looking results, consider getting expert advice if you decide to color your hair to conceal gray areas. Touch-ups may need to be done frequently.

3. Facial Hair: Men should maintain well-groomed, clipped facial hair. If you're a woman who would rather get rid of facial hair, you might want to look into threading, waxing, or laser hair removal.

4. Nail Care: Make sure your nails are neat and well-groomed. Ingrown nails can be avoided and a polished appearance can be maintained with regular manicures and pedicures.

5. Dental Care: Consistently clean and floss your teeth to maintain proper oral hygiene. If desired, think about getting dental work done, such as teeth whitening.

6. Wardrobe: Invest in new clothes that fit nicely and give you a confident appearance. Think of classic pieces that go well with your body   type   and   style.

7. Accessories: Sunglasses, jewelry, and scarves can all improve your appearance and lend an air of   sophistication.

8. Eyewear: If you wear glasses, pick styles and shapes of frames that go well with your face. Regularly changing your prescription will help you   maintain   optimal   vision.

9. Fragrance: Wear a delicate cologne or scent that complements your style without being too strong.

10. Confidence: The best part about grooming is having confidence. Accept the wisdom that comes with growing older and project confidence   in   your   own   skin. Recall that self-care is a personal journey, and that being at ease and self-assured in your own skin is the most crucial component. In order to make you look and feel your best as you embrace the age of 50 and beyond, skincare and grooming regimens should be customized to your individual preferences and demands.

7. chapter

WARDROBE AND FASHION

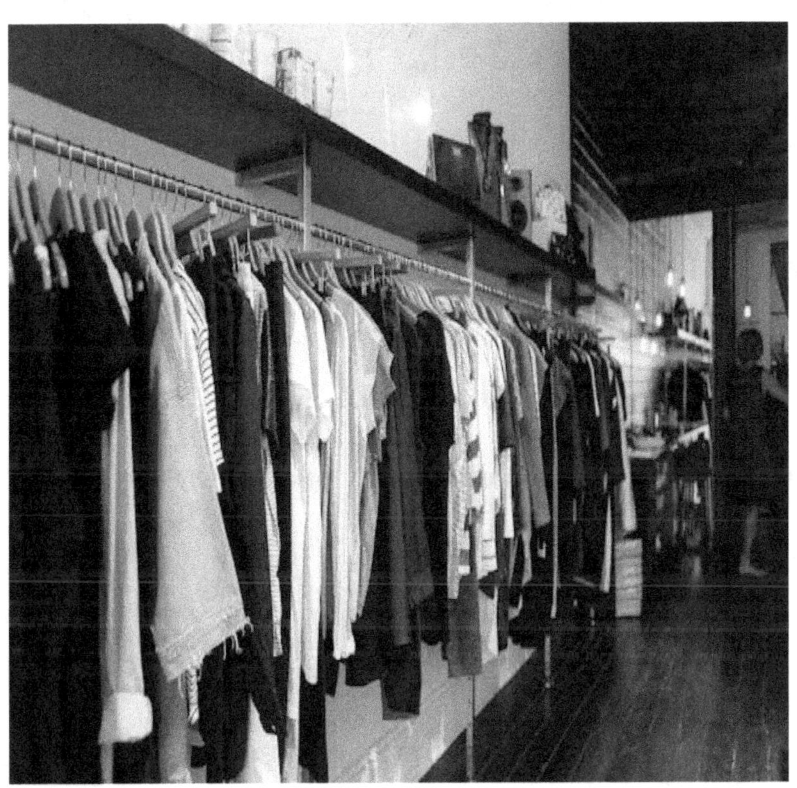

Fashion and wardrobe choices are statements of personal style that have a significant impact on how someone presents themselves and how confident they feel, particularly as people get older and older. The following are some pointers and things to think about when keeping an elegant and age-appropriate wardrobe:

1. Establish Your Style: Recognize your own tastes for classic, boho, modern, or eclectic looks. Understanding your personal style will enable you to dress with greater confidence and coherence.

2. Invest in Timeless Basics: Complement your wardrobe with well-made, classic pieces like well-fitting jeans, white shirts, blazers, and elegant gowns. These adaptable components can serve as the basis for many different looks.

3. Fit Matters: Make sure the clothes you wear fit properly. An important factor in determining how your clothes fit and seem on you is tailoring. Don't wear anything too tight or too loose.

4. Color Palette: Pick a color scheme that goes well with your skin tone and style. Although neutral colors like white, black, gray, and navy are adaptable choices, feel free to add color pops if that's how you want to style your space.

5. Mix & Match: To increase the number of ways you can wear an item, build a wardrobe that can be mixed and matched. As a result, you can wear your clothes for longer.

6. Comfort is Key: Give comfort top priority without compromising style. Choose materials that are comfortable next to your skin, and think about getting supportive shoes.

7. Declutter and Organize: Take regular inventory of your closet and get rid of anything you don't need or wear. Sort and arrange your clothes so that putting together outfits will be simpler.

8. Accessories: To give your outfits personality and flair, accessorise them with items like hats, jewelry, belts, and scarves. These can also be a reasonably priced approach to change the way you look.

9. Footwear: Make an investment in fashionable yet comfy shoes. For optimal foot health, take into account choices that offer support and cushioning.

10. Seasonal Wardrobe: To adjust to shifting weather patterns, maintain a seasonal wardrobe. To make room in your closet, store off-season apparel.

11. Pieces for Particular Occasions: Invest in a few pieces of clothing that are appropriate for different occasions, such as formal meetings, weddings, and parties. An exquisite dress or a well-fitting suit can be timeless purchases.

12. Undergarments: Make an investment in high-quality undergarments that provide your clothes the proper structure and support. Appropriate undergarments can enhance the comfort and fit of apparel.

13. Fashion Inspiration: Keep up with fashion-related blogs, journals, or social media pages that feature looks and trends that you find appealing. This may serve as motivation for your personal style decisions.

14. Eco-Friendly Decisions: Think about sustainable and environmentally friendly clothing selections. Select brands that use eco-friendly products and place a high priority on ethical production.

15. Confidence: In the end, self-assurance is the secret of outstanding fashion. Wear whatever suits your personality and makes you feel good. Accept the wisdom that comes with growing older.

16. Personal Grooming: Taking care of your skin, hair, and grooming habits goes a long way toward enhancing your overall appearance and matching your wardrobe selections. Keep in mind that there are no hard and fast rules when it comes to fashion—it's simply a method of self-expression. Your clothing should be a reflection of your lifestyle, comfort level, and personality. Use fashion as a tool to celebrate your individuality and show off your own style as you accept being over 50.

8. CHAPTER

SLEEP AND REST

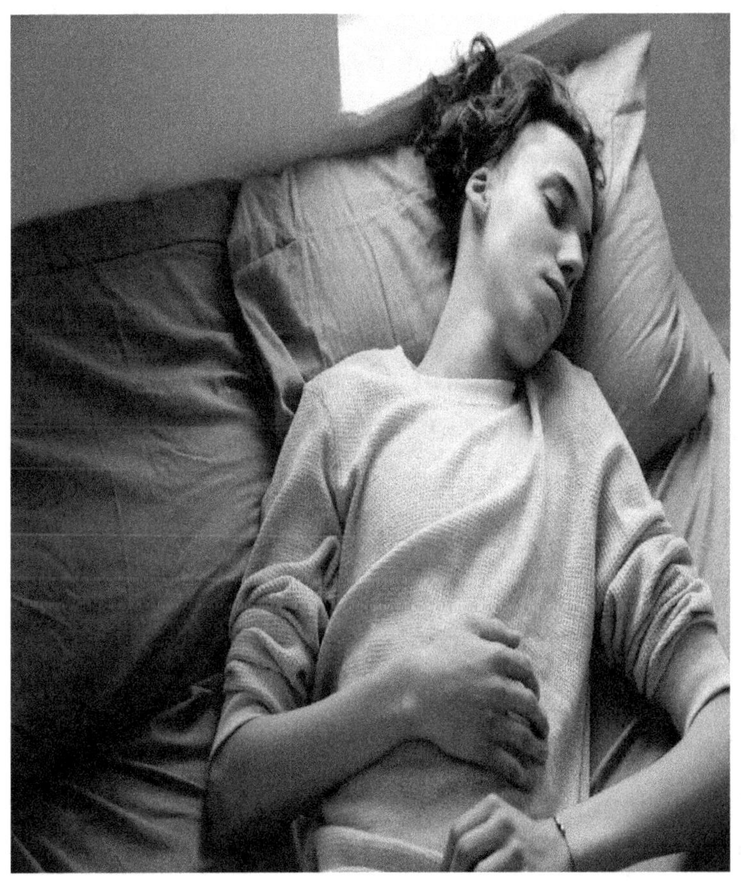

Good sleep and enough rest are vital for general health, especially when people get older than fifty years old. For mental clarity, emotional stability, physical health, and general vitality, sleep is essential. In order to maximize relaxation and sleep throughout this stage of life, keep the following points in mind:

1. **Make sleep hygiene a priority**. Even on weekends, set up a consistent sleep regimen by going to bed and waking up at the same times. Establish a cozy sleeping atmosphere by making sure your pillows and mattress are supportive, managing the temperature in the room, and reducing the amount of light and noise. If you're sleeping environment is not entirely dark, consider investing in blackout curtains or a sleep mask. Additionally, avoid using electronic gadgets in the bedroom as the blue light they create can disrupt your sleep. Avoid consuming too much alcohol and caffeine, especially after dark. Avoid eating heavy meals straight before bed.

2. **Reduce tension:** Before going to bed, try some relaxation methods like progressive

muscle relaxation, deep breathing, or meditation to reduce tension. To help you relax before bed, think about writing down any worries or concerns in a journal.

3. Exercise Frequently: Get moving on a regular basis, but steer clear of intense exercise right before bed because it can be stimulating. Yoga and other mild exercises can help you relax.

4. Limit Screen Time: At least one hour before going to bed, limit your exposure to screens, including those on computers, smartphones, and televisions. The natural sleep-wake cycle of your body may be disturbed by the blue light emitted by displays.

5. Pay Attention to What You Eat and Drink: Steer clear of heavy, spicy, or acidic foods right before bed because they can make you uncomfortable or induce indigestion. Minimize your nighttime fluid consumption to lessen the chance that you'll wake up in the middle of the night to use the restroom.

6. Handle Medication: Talk to your doctor about the time and any necessary adjustments if you take any medications that could interfere with your ability to sleep. Plan a peaceful before-bedtime ritual, such reading a book, having a warm bath, or doing light stretches.ϖ7. Establish a Calm Before Bedtime Routine:

8. **Seek Professional Help:** For an assessment and treatment alternatives, speak with a healthcare professional or sleep specialist if you frequently suffer from sleep disorders such insomnia, REM syndrome, or sleep apnea.

9. **Daytime Naps:** Despite the fact that quick naps throughout the day can be revitalizing, prolonged or late-afternoon naps should be avoided as they may disrupt sleep at night.

10. Listen to Your Body: - Be aware of the cues that your body gives you. Should you frequently experience fatigue throughout the day, it could be a sign that you require additional restorative sleep during the night.

11. **Keep Your Bedroom at a Comfortable Temperature:** Generally speaking, a room should be between 60 and 67 degrees

Fahrenheit (15 and 19 degrees Celsius) for sleeping.

12. Remain Active Throughout the Day: Getting regular exercise will help you sleep better. However, aim to work out earlier in the day rather than right before bed.

13. Limit Alcohol and Nicotine: Try to stay away from alcohol and nicotine, especially in the hours before bed, as these might interfere with sleep patterns.

Keep in mind that everyone has different demands when it comes to sleep, so it's critical to choose a schedule that suits you. Making sleep and rest a priority can have a big impact on your physical and mental health, enabling you to age with more health and vitality.

9. CHAPTER

PREVENTIVE HEALTHCARE

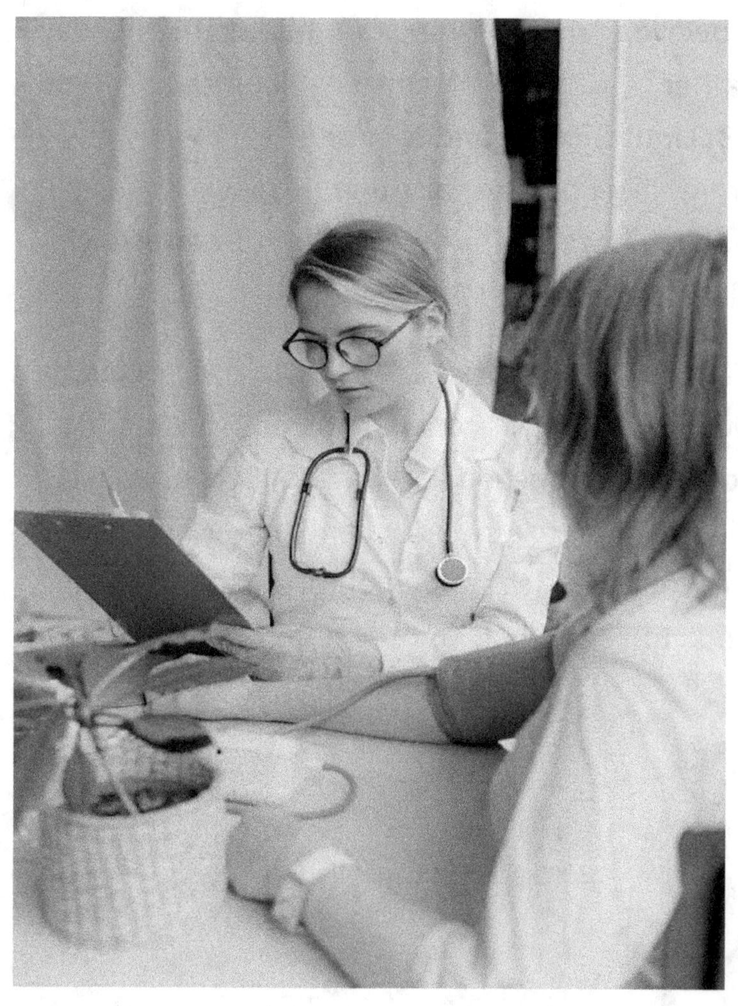

A vital component of preserving health and wellbeing is preventive healthcare, particularly as people get older (50 and beyond). Preventive care can lower the risk of chronic diseases, help identify and treat health issues early, and support an improved quality of life as people age. For this age range, the following are essential elements of preventative healthcare:

1. Frequent Health Check-Ups: Make an appointment with your primary care physician for regular check-ups. These checkups can provide a baseline for your medical history, assess your general health, and identify any new health issues.

2. Health Screenings: Adhere to suggested screening protocols for ailments like:

o Cancer: Based on your gender, family history, and risk factors, get regular screenings for breast, colorectal, prostate, and other cancers.

o **Heart disease:** ECGs, blood pressure measurements, cholesterol assessments, and other tests as necessary.

o **Diabetes:** If you have risk factors or a family history of the disease, get an A1c measurement and blood glucose test results.

o **Bone Health**: DXA scans for determining the risk of osteoporosis.

o **Vision and Eyes:** Routine eye exams to check for cataracts and glaucoma.

o **Hearing:** Hearing examinations as necessary to keep an eye on auditory wellness.

3. **Immunizations:** Make sure you get all the injections that are advised, such as the flu shot, the pneumonia vaccine, the shingles vaccine, and any additional doses that your doctor may recommend depending on your health and

travel   schedule.

4. Medication Management: Pay close attention to your doctor's recommendations if you take medication. Keep your healthcare staff informed of any changes in your health and raise any concerns you may have. Also, be mindful of possible interactions and adverse effects.

5. Healthy Lifestyle Options: Preserve a diet rich in fruits, vegetables, whole grains, lean meats, and healthy fats; keep it balanced. Regularly partake in physical activities appropriate for your level of fitness and capabilities.

Avoid smoking and consume alcohol in moderation.

Take up stress-relieving activities like yoga, meditation, or deep breathing.

6. Bone Health: To maintain bone health, make sure you're getting adequate calcium and vitamin D through diet and, if needed, supplements.

Weight-bearing activities can support the preservation of bone density.

7. Vision and Hearing Care: Keep up with routine eye and hearing tests to keep an eye on changes in your vision and hearing, and take quick action to remedy any problems.

8. Mental Health: Be mindful of your emotional and mental health. If you are experiencing signs of depression, anxiety, or other mental health issues, get professional assistance.

9. Dental Health: Ensure proper dental hygiene by consistently brushing and flossing. Make time for routine dental cleanings and examinations.

10. Skin Health: - Examine your own skin for changes and irregularities, and see a dermatologist if you find any suspicious lesions or moles.

11. Remain Informed: - Keep yourself updated on medical developments and health-related topics. Continue to be involved in your medical decisions and speak out for your needs.

12. Prevent Falls: - Take preventive measures to avoid falling, like keeping your home clutter-free, utilizing handrails, and exercising frequently to strengthen and balance yourself.

13. Know Your Family History: - Genetics can greatly influence your likelihood of developing certain disorders, therefore it's important to be informed of your family's medical history. Talk about this with your medical professional.

14. Social Engagement:- As social engagement

has been connected to improved general health and well-being, continue to be socially engaged and cultivate good relationships. You may lower your risk of various health issues and increase your chances of living a long, healthy, and active life as you age by actively taking part in preventative healthcare practices. To create a customized preventive healthcare plan based on your unique requirements and risk factors, speak with your healthcare practitioner.

10. CHAPTER

STAYING SOCIALLY CONNECTED

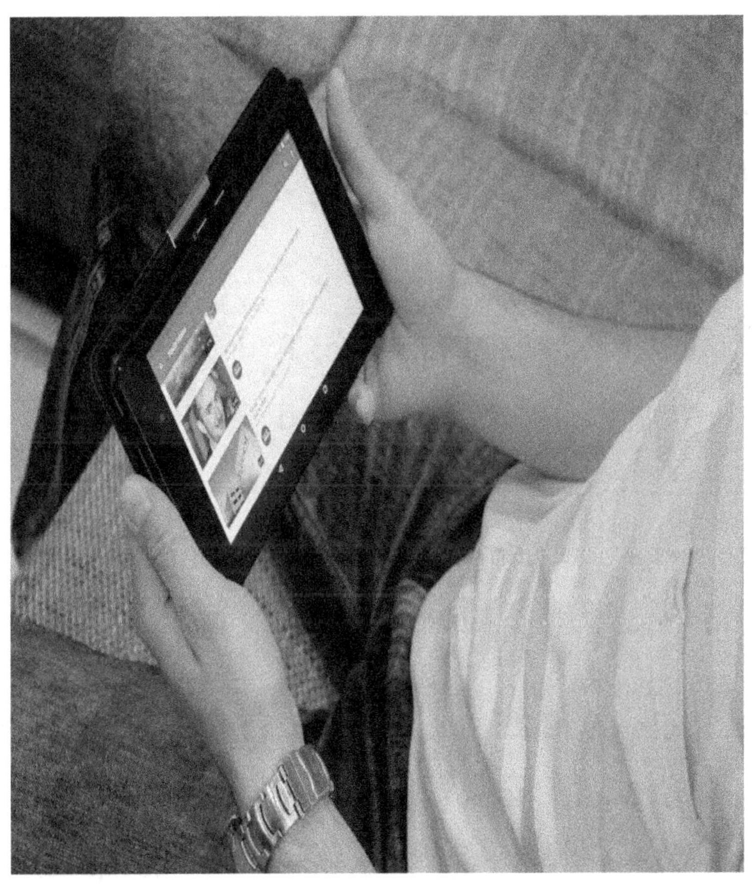

Maintaining social connections is essential to living a happy and healthy life, particularly as people get older (over 50). Emotional health, cognitive function, and general quality of life are all influenced by social contacts, relationships, and community involvement. The following are some methods for maintaining social connections:

1. ties should be prioritized: Take care of your current ties with friends and family. Try to maintain contact as often as you can by phone conversations, emails, video chats, or in-person meetings.

2. Join Social Groups: Look for regional associations, clubs, or interest-based groups that share your interests or passions. Participating in book clubs, gardening clubs, or sports leagues might offer chances to connect with people who share similar interests.

3. Volunteer: Engaging in volunteer work for a cause you are passionate about not only enables you to give back to the community but also gives you a feeling of direction and a way to connect with like-minded individuals.

4. Attend Community Events: Take part in neighborhood get-togethers, fairs, and festivals. These events can be fantastic chances to interact with your community and meet new people.

5. Attend Classes or Workshops: Sign up for workshops or classes that pique your interest, such as attending educational lectures, picking up a creative activity, or learning a new language. These environments foster interpersonal communication and personal development.

6. Make Use of Technology: Using social media, messaging applications, and video calls, you may stay in touch with friends and relatives who live far away.

7. Visit Senior Centers: Senior centers can provide a variety of activities, such as arts and crafts and exercise programs, in many towns. These facilities might offer a welcoming setting for mingling with other students.

8. Explore and Travel: Traveling, whether domestically or abroad, can offer chances to meet new people and take in various cultures. Take into account senior-focused excursions or travel groups.

Get in touch with friends from your previous school or university years. Maintaining social connections through rekindling old friendships can be fulfilling.

9. Reestablish Contact with Old Friends:

Make contact with pals from your past, including those from college or high school. Maintaining social connections through rekindling old friendships can be fulfilling.

10. Participate in Religious or Spiritual Gatherings: - If you identify as religious or spiritual, attending events at your local mosque, church, or synagogue can foster a strong sense of belonging.

11. Listen Well: - Engage in active listening when interacting with people. Being genuinely interested in their experiences and tales can help your relationships grow.

12. Promote Intergenerational Relationships: - Engage in activities with younger generations, such neighborhood youth organizations or grandchildren. These exchanges can give both parties a sense of purpose and enrichment.

13. Seek expert Help: Don't be afraid to ask a mental health expert or counselor for assistance if you're struggling with social isolation, loneliness, or mental health issues.

14. Be Open to New Experiences: - Seize the chance to meet people from different backgrounds and to experience new things. Increasing your social circle might result in enlightening viewpoints and experiences.

15. Plan Social activities: - Take the initiative to schedule get-togethers, activities, or outings with friends and family. Having the role of host can make one feel fulfilled and connected.

Maintaining social connections involves both the volume and quality of encounters. Develop deep connections with others and partake in pursuits that make you happy and fulfilled. As you get older, having social ties might improve your emotional and mental health.

11. CHAPTER

EMBRACING HOBBIES AND INTERESTS

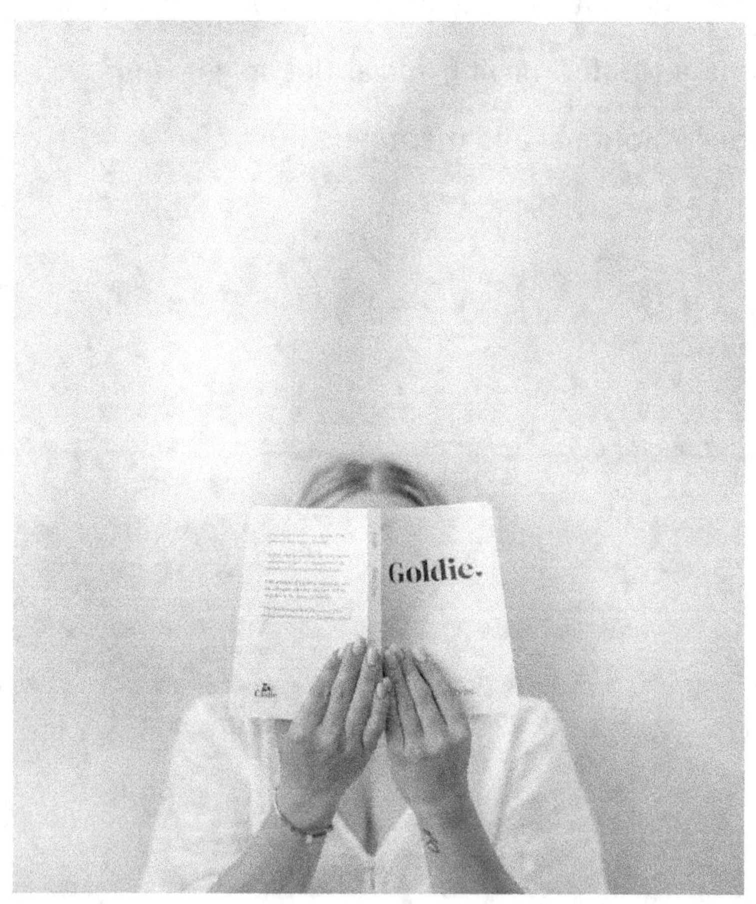

Taking up interests and hobbies is a rewarding and enriching part of life, particularly for people who are 50 years of age and older. These pursuits offer chances for social interaction, creativity, leisure, and personal development. Here are several justifications for this as well as advice on embracing interests and hobbies as you age:

Reasons to Welcome Interests and Hobbies:

1. Personal Fulfillment: Interests and hobbies can lead to a sense of personal fulfillment. Taking part in pursuits that you are enthusiastic about might make you feel happy and accomplished.

2. Stress Reduction: Hobbies give people a way to decompress. Getting lost in your favorite activity can ease anxiety and encourage calm.

3. Mental Stimulation: A variety of pastimes

stimulate the mind and promote lifelong learning. Preventing cognitive deterioration and preserving mental acuity can be achieved through this cognitive activity.

4. Physical Activity: Engaging in physical activities as a hobby, such as dance, gardening, or sports, can improve your general health and wellbeing.

5. Social Interaction: Engaging in hobbies can result in meeting new people. You can meet people who share your interests by signing up for organizations, groups, or classes.

6. Creativity: Whether it's writing, painting, or creating, hobbies frequently have a creative component. Being creative may be a very effective way to express oneself.

7. Sense of Purpose: Hobbies, particularly if you're retired or have more leisure time, provide your everyday life structure and a sense of purpose.

Advice for Embracing Interests and Hobbies:

1. Consider Your Interests: Think about the pursuits or hobbies that have always piqued your curiosity or that you've wanted to investigate. Think about your passions and the things that make you happy.

2. Start Small: Don't feel obligated to become an expert in a new pastime right away. Build your abilities and knowledge gradually, starting with modest, doable stages.

3. Set Achievable Goals: Make realistic goals according to your pastime. Setting goals can help you stay motivated, whether it's finishing a book, painting, or learning a new cuisine. Establish a Dedicated Space: If your interest calls for a certain section of your house, set aside a room where you may practice it comfortably.

5. Attend seminars or Classes: To improve your abilities and meet people who share your interests, sign up for seminars or classes linked to your passion.

6. Join Clubs or Groups: Look for internet forums or local clubs dedicated to your interest. Having conversations with people who share your interests might be beneficial.

7. Maintain Balance in Your Hobbies: Having a variety of hobbies is wonderful, but keep things in check. Make sure you have adequate time for all of your interests and other significant responsibilities.

8. Be Open to Trying New Things: Keep an Open Mind on Hobbies and Interests. Experimentation can reveal hidden passions and promote human development.

9. Practice Often: The secret to getting better at any pastime is consistency. Set aside time each day to practice or participate in the activity of your choice.

10. Accept the Learning Process: Recognize that pursuing your interests may provide obstacles and disappointments. Accept these as chances for personal development.

11. Share Your Hobbies: Talk about your interests with loved ones and invite them to join you in your hobbies. It might be a fostering moment.

12. Adapt as Needed: As you get older and your interests and physical capabilities change, be adaptable and open to modify your hobbies. Taking up interests and hobbies is a lifetime journey that can provide happiness, contentment, and a feeling of direction. No matter your age, discovering new interests and following your passions can improve your general wellbeing and enrich your life.

12. CHAPTER

PLANNING FOR THE FUTURE

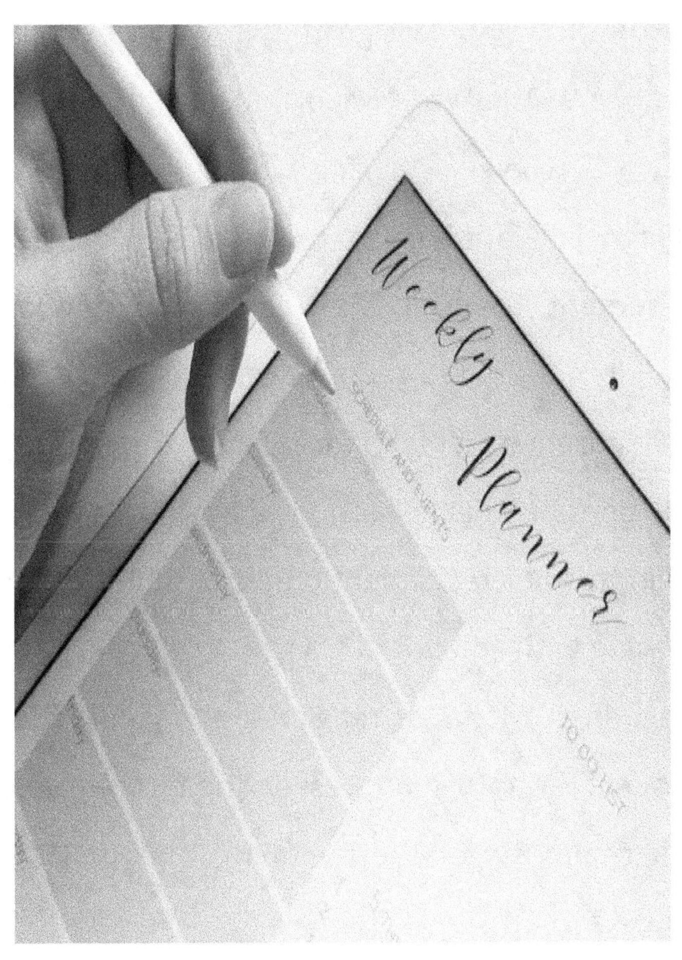

Making plans for the future is an essential part of living, particularly for those who are 50 years of age and beyond. A well-thought-out plan can provide you peace of mind, financial security, and the power to design the life you desire in later years. These are important things to think about when making future plans:

1. Financial Planning:

Retirement Savings: Make sure you have a carefully considered retirement strategy. Assess your retirement assets, including 401(k)s, IRAs, and pension plans; for advice on how to maximize your retirement portfolio, think about speaking with a financial advisor.

Budgeting: Make a reasonable budget that accounts for both your present and future costs, such as housing, entertainment, and medical care. If you want to become financially stable, follow your budget.

Estate Planning: Take into account drafting or revising your estate plan, which should include powers of attorney, trusts, and wills. By doing this, you can reduce the possibility of legal issues for your loved ones and guarantee that your assets are dispersed in accordance with your preferences.

Examine your alternatives for long-term care insurance to safeguard your assets and meet your care requirements in the event of a sickness or incapacity.

Healthcare Planning: Arrange for the medical care you will require, such as screenings, preventive care, and routine checkups. To express your medical wishes, think about creating advance directives or healthcare proxies.

2. Health and Wellness: Make a healthy lifestyle a priority, incorporating exercise, a balanced diet, and effective stress management to enhance general health and lower the likelihood of chronic ailments. Housing Options: Assess your present living arrangement and determine whether it satisfies your needs over the long run. Examine choices including assisted living, senior communities, downsizing, and aging in place adaptations. Location: Think about where you want to live in the future, keeping in mind things like accessibility to family, medical facilities, and amenities that improve your quality of life.

3. Housing and Living Arrangements: Legal Records: Make sure you have a living will, durable power of attorney, healthcare proxy, and other necessary legal documents in place.

4. End-of-life and Legal Planning: Plans for the Funeral and Burial: Tell your loved ones about any particular funeral or burial choices you may have, and make the necessary preparations ahead of time.

Social ties: Sustain and grow your relationships with others. Make time for hobbies, get-togethers with friends and family, and social events.

5. Emotional and Social Welfare: Mental Health: Be mindful of your mental well-being and, if necessary, seek expert assistance. Mental wellness is essential to overall well being.

6. Legacy and Giving:

 Legacy Planning: Think about your legacy and your desired memory. Consider making gifts to charities, engaging in philanthropic activities, or transferring family customs and values.

7. Lifelong Learning and Personal Development: Take advantage of possibilities for ongoing education and development. Ongoing intellectual stimulation is crucial, whether it comes from reading, learning new things, or taking classes.

8. Flexibility and Adaptability: Make a Change Management Plan: Acknowledge that plans may need to be modified because life is unpredictable. Retain an open mind and be ready to adjust as situations change.

9. Seek Expert Advice: Consult Subject Matter Experts: To make sure your plans are thorough and in line with your objectives, don't be afraid to consult experts in the fields of finance, estate planning, healthcare, and law. Recall that future planning is a continuous endeavor. As your needs, objectives, and situation change over time, revisit and revise your plans on a regular basis. Making the most of your latter years can bring you peace of mind and proactive planning for the future.

13. CHAPTER

REAL-LIFE SUCCESS STORIES

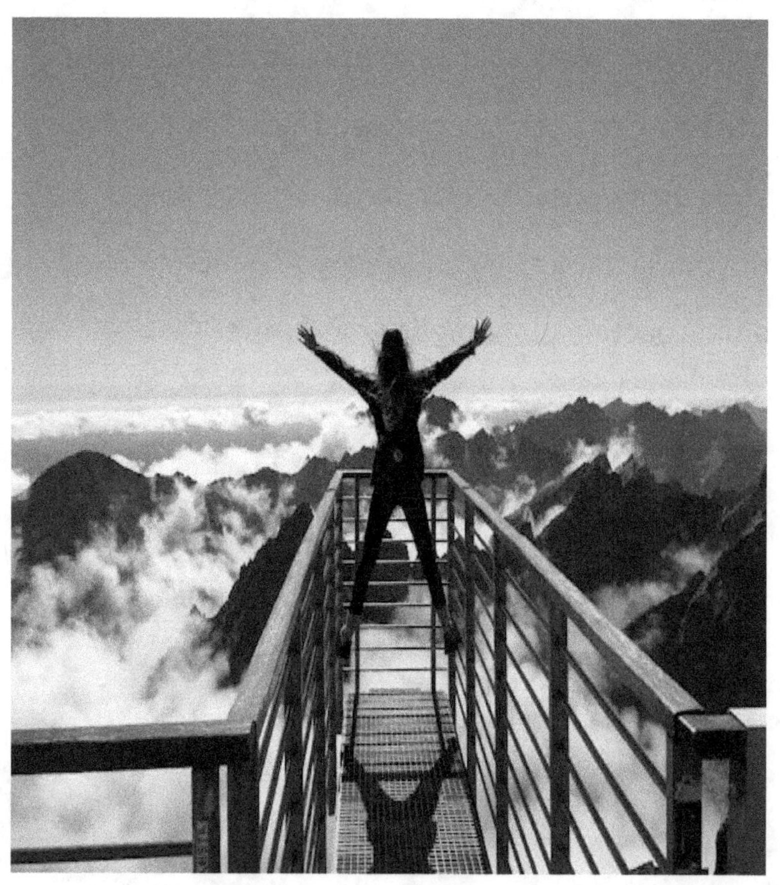

Of course! Here are a few true success stories of people who, after turning 50, accomplished amazing   feats:

1. Vera Wang, Fashion Designer: Vera Wang began her career in fashion design at the age of forty-nine. She started out at Vogue as an editor before moving on to Ralph Lauren as a design director. She became one of the most well-known bridal gown designers in the world when she launched her own bridal boutique at the age of 40.

2. Colonel Sanders (KFC Founder): At the age of sixty-two, Harland Sanders, better known as Colonel Sanders, started Kentucky Fried Chicken (KFC). He remained the brand's ambassador and spokesperson even after selling his franchise and   recipe.

3. Laura Ingalls Wilder, Author: Although she wrote the adored "Little House on the Prairie" series, Laura Ingalls Wilder didn't begin writing until she was in her late 40s. Since then, her works have been widely read by children and have been turned into a hit television series.

4. Ray Kroc, the McDonald brothers' founder: Ray Kroc met the brothers when he was in his 50s and helped grow their little fast-food joint into the international success it is today.

5. Julia Child, Chef and TV Personality: Julia Child didn't begin her profession in cooking until she was in her late 30s, when she enrolled at Paris's Cordon Bleu culinary school. Her subsequent contributions to television culinary shows and cookbook writing transformed American cooking.

6. Stan Lee (Comic Book Creator): In his 40s and 50s, Stan Lee collaborated on the creation of well-known comic book characters like Spider-Man, the X-Men, Iron Man, and the Fantastic Four. His contributions to the entertainment industry have had a significant influence.

7. Anna Mary Robertson Moses (Grandma Moses, Artist): At the age of 78, Anna Mary Robertson Moses started painting. Her paintings of folk art brought her fame, and they are currently on exhibit in museums all over the world.

8. Sam Walton, the company's founder: At the age of 44, Sam Walton set up the company's first store. He went on to establish an empire in retail that grew to become one of the biggest and most prosperous businesses in the world. These true success stories demonstrate how age need never be a hindrance to following one's passions, launching new businesses, or accomplishing noteworthy goals. They serve as a reminder that it's never too late to pursue our goals and change the world for the better.

SUMMARY ON HOW TO LOOK MORE HEALTHY AT 50

I'm not familiar with any particular books or their contents, but I can give you a broad rundown of the essential ideas for looking and feeling better at fifty:

1. Put nutrition first: Eating a nutritious, well-balanced diet full of whole grains, fruits, vegetables, lean meats, and healthy fats is crucial to sustaining good health. Pay attention to portion quantities and be properly hydrated.

2. Regular Exercise: Take part in regular physical activity that incorporates strength training and cardiovascular exercise. This promotes the preservation of bone density, muscle mass, and general fitness.

3. Good Sleep: Make sure you obtain adequate restorative sleep every night. Create a cozy sleeping space, stick to a regular sleep routine, and follow proper sleep hygiene.

4. Skin Care: Establish a regimen that consists of exfoliation, hydration, and SPF protection. Make use of items suitable for your age and skin type.

5. Hydration: To keep your body and skin hydrated, drink lots of water. Consuming too much alcohol or coffee might cause dehydration.

6. Stress Management: To effectively manage stress, engage in stress-reduction practices like deep breathing exercises, yoga, meditation, or mindfulness.

7. Regular Health Check-ups: Make an appointment with your healthcare provider on a regular basis to discuss any concerns you may have about your health as well as to receive immunizations and preventive health screenings.

8. Social Networks: Sustain and grow your social networks. Maintaining relationships with friends and family is essential for mental health.

9. Mental Health: Give your mental well-being some thought. If you require medical attention for illnesses like sadness or anxiety, do so.

10. Hobbies and Interests: Take part in pursuits that you find inspiring. Engaging in hobbies can lead to both mental and emotional fulfillment.

11. Regular Dental and Eye Care: Take good care of your teeth and eyes. Checkups on a regular basis can help identify and treat problems early.

12. Grooming and Wardrobe: Wear clothing that accentuates your sense of self-worth and comfort. Consider personal hygiene and grooming.

13. Positive Thinking: Keep an optimistic perspective on life. Practice thankfulness and concentrate on the things that make you happy and fulfilled.

14. Minimize Dangerous Habits: As they can negatively impact one's beauty and health, reduce or give up bad habits like smoking and binge drinking.

15. Remain Informed: Learn about the aging process and any particular health issues that can surface with age. Acquiring knowledge gives one strength.

16. Adaptability: Have an open mind and learn to work with the aging process. Accept the wisdom that comes with growing older. Keep in mind that every person's path to looking and feeling well at 50 is different. These guidelines offer a broad framework, but it's crucial to modify your strategy to fit your unique requirements and situation. Seeking advice from specialists and healthcare professionals can offer tailored direction towards achieving maximum health and wellness.

www.ingramcontent.com/pod-product-compliance
Lightning Source LLC
Chambersburg PA
CBHW051828250726
48659CB00005B/1723